Fitness Journal
My Goals, My Training, and My Success

Fitness Journal
My Goals, My Training, and My Success

Karen M. Goeller

Fitness Journal

My Goals, My Training, and My Success

Before starting any exercise program discuss it with your doctor or medical professional.

My Goals, My Training, and My Success

Congratulations on making the decision to keep track of your fitness training and daily food intake.

Whether you are just beginning to take on a new exercise routine or you've been working out and eating healthy foods for several years, keeping a journal is a great way to set goals and track your health related habits.

Months from now you will have the opportunity to see how well you have reached your fitness goals or made healthy changes in your diet.

This journal will be a record of the methods you used to reach your fitness and nutritional goals.

Maybe the goals will be reached or maybe they will be changed, but at the very least you will have documented important lifestyle changes and activities.

Remember to always keep safety in mind when performing any exercise routine and be sure to choose healthy foods while preparing your meals and snacks.

Best of luck reaching your fitness goals!

Before starting any exercise program discuss it with your doctor or medical professional.

My Goals, My Training, and My Success

Fitness Journal 5
My Goals, My Training, and My Success

Name___________________________**Age**________**Date**__________

Fitness Trainer or Workout Partner__________________________________
Weight_________Percent Body Fat________Blood Pressure___________
Resting Heart Rate____________Target Heart Rate___________________
Medications____
____
Medical Problems____
____

Current Fitness Level
Never Exercise / Exercise Occasionally / Weekend Athlete / Exercise
Often / Competitive Athlete / High Fitness Level

____
____

What motivated me to begin a steady exercise program?
Doctor / Health Issues / Upcoming Event / Stress / Social Reasons

____
____
____

Long Term Fitness Goals
Weight Loss / Sculpt Body / Strength / Sports Specific / Health

____
____
____

3 Month Fitness Goals

____
____
____

1 Month Fitness Goals

____
____
____

I plan to exercise ________ days each week.

____

Before starting any exercise program discuss it with your doctor or medical professional.

My Goals, My Training, and My Success

How am I going to avoid distraction during workout today?

____

____

Goal for Today's Workout
Cardiovascular / Weight or Repetitions / Focus / Exercise Form / Other

____

____

____

____

What did I eat and drink before today's workout?

____

____

____

____

How do I feel before today's workout?
Energized / Motivated / Content / Drained / Exhausted / Unmotivated

____

____

Fitness Journal
My Goals, My Training, and My Success

Strength Exercise Chart		
	Resistance	
	Repetitions	
	Sets	
	Resistance	
	Repetitions	
	Sets	
	Resistance	
	Repetitions	
	Sets	
	Resistance	
	Repetitions	
	Sets	
	Resistance	
	Repetitions	
	Sets	
	Resistance	
	Repetitions	
	Sets	
	Resistance	
	Repetitions	
	Sets	
	Resistance	
	Repetitions	
	Sets	
	Resistance	
	Repetitions	
	Sets	
Cardiovascular Exercise		
	Time	
	Time	
Stretching Exercise		
	Hold Time	
	Hold Time	
	Hold Time	
	Hold Time	

Before starting any exercise program discuss it with your doctor or medical professional.

Fitness Journal
My Goals, My Training, and My Success

Did I reach my goal for today?______________________

____

____

How do I feel at end of today's workout?
Energized / Motivated / Content / Drained / Exhausted / Disappointed

____

____

____

Goals for next workout:_______________________

____

____

____

Fitness Trainer's suggestions for next workout:______

____

____

____

Most recent advice from Health Care Professional
Health Status / Goals / Fitness Commitment

____

____

____

____

Were there any injuries or illnesses before or during today's workout?______________________________

____

____

____

My Goals, My Training, and My Success

Nutritional Section

A great way to discover whether you are getting all of the nutrients your body needs is to write down everything you eat for one week. Once you have the list compare the nutrient values in the foods you have consumed to the nutrient values recommended by your doctor or the recommended dietary allowance. Discuss the results with your doctor or other medical professional in order to improve or maintain your health.

Many people use a chart system similar to this one.

Food	Protein	Vit A	Vit D	Vit E	Vit K	Vit C	Thiamin B1	Riboflavin B2	Niacin B3	Iron	Calcium
Breakfast											
Snack											
Lunch											
Snack											
Dinner											
Snack											
Totals											

Food Consumed Today

Breakfast____

Snack____

Lunch____

Snack____
Dinner____

Snack____

Fitness Journal 10
My Goals, My Training, and My Success

Motivation for eating healthy:_________________________
____
____
____

Immediate nutritional goals:__________________________
____
____
____

Did I meet my nutritional goals today?_________________
____
____

Long term nutritional or health related goals:_________
____
____
____

What changes in nutrition are necessary?
Increase Fluid Intake / Increase Fiber Intake / Decrease Unhealthy Foods / Decrease Unhealthy Beverages / Increase Fruits or Vegetables / Increase Vitamin or Mineral____
____
____
____
____

Recent advice from doctor or other medical professional regarding nutrition:_______________________________
____
____
____

Was it difficult to follow the nutritional advice from my doctor or medical professional?___________________
____

Before starting any exercise program discuss it with your doctor or medical professional.

Fitness Journal
My Goals, My Training, and My Success

My thoughts:

Fitness Journal
My Goals, My Training, and My Success

Fitness Journal
My Goals, My Training, and My Success

Name_______________________________**Age**_________**Date**__________

Fitness Trainer or Workout Partner______________________________
Weight_________Percent Body Fat_________Blood Pressure___________
Resting Heart Rate____________Target Heart Rate___________________
Medications____
____
Medical Problems____
____

Current Fitness Level
Never Exercise / Exercise Occasionally / Weekend Athlete / Exercise
Often / Competitive Athlete / High Fitness Level

____
____

What motivated me to begin a steady exercise program?
Doctor / Health Issues / Upcoming Event / Stress / Social Reasons

____
____
____

Long Term Fitness Goals
Weight Loss / Sculpt Body / Strength / Sports Specific / Health

____
____
____

3 Month Fitness Goals

____
____
____

1 Month Fitness Goals

____
____
____

I plan to exercise _______ days each week.

____

Before starting any exercise program discuss it with your doctor or medical professional.

My Goals, My Training, and My Success

How am I going to avoid distraction during workout today?

____

____

Goal for Today's Workout
Cardiovascular / Weight or Repetitions / Focus / Exercise Form / Other

____

____

____

____

What did I eat and drink before today's workout?

____

____

____

____

How do I feel before today's workout?
Energized / Motivated / Content / Drained / Exhausted / Unmotivated

____

____

My Goals, My Training, and My Success

Strength Exercise Chart		
	Resistance	
	Repetitions	
	Sets	
	Resistance	
	Repetitions	
	Sets	
	Resistance	
	Repetitions	
	Sets	
	Resistance	
	Repetitions	
	Sets	
	Resistance	
	Repetitions	
	Sets	
	Resistance	
	Repetitions	
	Sets	
	Resistance	
	Repetitions	
	Sets	
	Resistance	
	Repetitions	
	Sets	
	Resistance	
	Repetitions	
	Sets	
Cardiovascular Exercise		
	Time	
	Time	
Stretching Exercise		
	Hold Time	
	Hold Time	
	Hold Time	
	Hold Time	

Before starting any exercise program discuss it with your doctor or medical professional.

Fitness Journal
My Goals, My Training, and My Success

Did I reach my goal for today?____________________
____

____

How do I feel at end of today's workout?
Energized / Motivated / Content / Drained / Exhausted / Disappointed

____

____

____

Goals for next workout:____________________________
____

____

____

Fitness Trainer's suggestions for next workout:________
____

____

____

Most recent advice from Health Care Professional
Health Status / Goals / Fitness Commitment

____

____

____

____

Were there any injuries or illnesses before or during today's workout?________________________________
____

____

____

My Goals, My Training, and My Success

Nutritional Section

A great way to discover whether you are getting all of the nutrients your body needs is to write down everything you eat for one week. Once you have the list compare the nutrient values in the foods you have consumed to the nutrient values recommended by your doctor or the recommended dietary allowance. Discuss the results with your doctor or other medical professional in order to improve or maintain your health.

Many people use a chart system similar to this one.

Food	Protein	Vit A	Vit D	Vit E	Vit K	Vit C	Thiamin B1	Riboflavin B2	Niacin B3	Iron	Calcium
Breakfast											
Snack											
Lunch											
Snack											
Dinner											
Snack											
Totals											

Food Consumed Today

Breakfast____

____

Snack____

____

Lunch____

____

____

____

Snack____
Dinner____

____

____

____

Snack____

Fitness Journal
My Goals, My Training, and My Success

Motivation for eating healthy:_______________________

____

____

____

Immediate nutritional goals:_______________________

____

____

____

Did I meet my nutritional goals today?_______________

____

____

Long term nutritional or health related goals:__________

____

____

____

What changes in nutrition are necessary?
Increase Fluid Intake / Increase Fiber Intake / Decrease Unhealthy Foods / Decrease Unhealthy Beverages / Increase Fruits or Vegetables / Increase Vitamin or Mineral_______________________________________

____

____

____

____

Recent advice from doctor or other medical professional regarding nutrition:_______________________

____

____

____

Was it difficult to follow the nutritional advice from my doctor or medical professional?_______________

____

Before starting any exercise program discuss it with your doctor or medical professional.

Fitness Journal

My Goals, My Training, and My Success

My thoughts:

Fitness Journal
My Goals, My Training, and My Success

Fitness Journal

My Goals, My Training, and My Success

Name_______________________________**Age**_________**Date**__________

Fitness Trainer or Workout Partner_________________________________
Weight_________Percent Body Fat_________Blood Pressure___________
Resting Heart Rate_____________Target Heart Rate___________________
Medications____
____
Medical Problems____
____

Current Fitness Level

Never Exercise / Exercise Occasionally / Weekend Athlete / Exercise Often / Competitive Athlete / High Fitness Level

____

____

What motivated me to begin a steady exercise program?

Doctor / Health Issues / Upcoming Event / Stress / Social Reasons

____

____

____

Long Term Fitness Goals

Weight Loss / Sculpt Body / Strength / Sports Specific / Health

____

____

____

3 Month Fitness Goals

____

____

____

1 Month Fitness Goals

____

____

____

I plan to exercise _______ days each week.

____

Before starting any exercise program discuss it with your doctor or medical professional.

How am I going to avoid distraction during workout today?

____

____

Goal for Today's Workout

Cardiovascular / Weight or Repetitions / Focus / Exercise Form / Other

____

____

____

____

What did I eat and drink before today's workout?

____

____

____

____

How do I feel before today's workout?

Energized / Motivated / Content / Drained / Exhausted / Unmotivated

____

____

Fitness Journal
My Goals, My Training, and My Success

Strength Exercise Chart	
	Resistance
	Repetitions
	Sets
	Resistance
	Repetitions
	Sets
	Resistance
	Repetitions
	Sets
	Resistance
	Repetitions
	Sets
	Resistance
	Repetitions
	Sets
	Resistance
	Repetitions
	Sets
	Resistance
	Repetitions
	Sets
	Resistance
	Repetitions
	Sets
	Resistance
	Repetitions
	Sets
Cardiovascular Exercise	
	Time
	Time
Stretching Exercise	
	Hold Time
	Hold Time
	Hold Time
	Hold Time

Before starting any exercise program discuss it with your doctor or medical professional.

Fitness Journal
My Goals, My Training, and My Success

Did I reach my goal for today?______________________

____

____

How do I feel at end of today's workout?
Energized / Motivated / Content / Drained / Exhausted / Disappointed

____

____

____

Goals for next workout:______________________

____

____

____

Fitness Trainer's suggestions for next workout:________

____

____

____

Most recent advice from Health Care Professional
Health Status / Goals / Fitness Commitment

____

____

____

____

Were there any injuries or illnesses before or during today's workout?______________________

____

____

____

My Goals, My Training, and My Success

Nutritional Section

A great way to discover whether you are getting all of the nutrients your body needs is to write down everything you eat for one week. Once you have the list compare the nutrient values in the foods you have consumed to the nutrient values recommended by your doctor or the recommended dietary allowance. Discuss the results with your doctor or other medical professional in order to improve or maintain your health.

Many people use a chart system similar to this one.

Food	Protein	Vit A	Vit D	Vit E	Vit K	Vit C	Thiamin B1	Riboflavin B2	Niacin B3	Iron	Calcium
Breakfast											
Snack											
Lunch											
Snack											
Dinner											
Snack											
Totals											

Food Consumed Today

Breakfast____

____

Snack____

____

Lunch____

____

____

Snack____
Dinner____

____

____

Snack____

Before starting any exercise program discuss it with your doctor or medical professional.

My Goals, My Training, and My Success

Motivation for eating healthy:______________________

____

____

____

Immediate nutritional goals:______________________

____

____

____

Did I meet my nutritional goals today?______________

____

____

Long term nutritional or health related goals:________

____

____

____

What changes in nutrition are necessary?
Increase Fluid Intake / Increase Fiber Intake / Decrease Unhealthy Foods /
Decrease Unhealthy Beverages / Increase Fruits or Vegetables / Increase Vitamin
or Mineral______________________________________

____

____

____

**Recent advice from doctor or other medical professional
regarding nutrition:**______________________________

____

____

**Was it difficult to follow the nutritional advice from my
doctor or medical professional?**____________________

____

Before starting any exercise program discuss it with your doctor or medical professional.

My Goals, My Training, and My Success

My thoughts:____

Fitness Journal
My Goals, My Training, and My Success

Fitness Journal 29

My Goals, My Training, and My Success

Name________________________________**Age**________**Date**__________

Fitness Trainer or Workout Partner_________________________________
Weight________Percent Body Fat________Blood Pressure__________
Resting Heart Rate____________Target Heart Rate__________________
Medications____

Medical Problems____
____

Current Fitness Level
Never Exercise / Exercise Occasionally / Weekend Athlete / Exercise
Often / Competitive Athlete / High Fitness Level

____

____

What motivated me to begin a steady exercise program?
Doctor / Health Issues / Upcoming Event / Stress / Social Reasons

____

____

____

Long Term Fitness Goals
Weight Loss / Sculpt Body / Strength / Sports Specific / Health

____

____

____

3 Month Fitness Goals

____

____

____

1 Month Fitness Goals

____

____

____

I plan to exercise _______ days each week.

____

My Goals, My Training, and My Success

How am I going to avoid distraction during workout today?

____

____

Goal for Today's Workout
Cardiovascular / Weight or Repetitions / Focus / Exercise Form / Other

____

____

____

____

What did I eat and drink before today's workout?

____

____

____

____

How do I feel before today's workout?
Energized / Motivated / Content / Drained / Exhausted / Unmotivated

____

____

Fitness Journal
My Goals, My Training, and My Success

Strength Exercise Chart	
	Resistance
	Repetitions
	Sets
	Resistance
	Repetitions
	Sets
	Resistance
	Repetitions
	Sets
	Resistance
	Repetitions
	Sets
	Resistance
	Repetitions
	Sets
	Resistance
	Repetitions
	Sets
	Resistance
	Repetitions
	Sets
	Resistance
	Repetitions
	Sets
	Resistance
	Repetitions
	Sets
Cardiovascular Exercise	
	Time
	Time
Stretching Exercise	
	Hold Time
	Hold Time
	Hold Time
	Hold Time

Before starting any exercise program discuss it with your doctor or medical professional.

Fitness Journal

My Goals, My Training, and My Success

Did I reach my goal for today?______________________

____

____

How do I feel at end of today's workout?
Energized / Motivated / Content / Drained / Exhausted / Disappointed

____

____

____

Goals for next workout:______________________________

____

____

____

Fitness Trainer's suggestions for next workout:________

____

____

____

Most recent advice from Health Care Professional
Health Status / Goals / Fitness Commitment

____

____

____

____

Were there any injuries or illnesses before or during today's workout?______________________________________

____

____

____

Before starting any exercise program discuss it with your doctor or medical professional.

My Goals, My Training, and My Success

Nutritional Section

A great way to discover whether you are getting all of the nutrients your body needs is to write down everything you eat for one week. Once you have the list compare the nutrient values in the foods you have consumed to the nutrient values recommended by your doctor or the recommended dietary allowance. Discuss the results with your doctor or other medical professional in order to improve or maintain your health.

Many people use a chart system similar to this one.

Food	Protein	Vit A	Vit D	Vit E	Vit K	Vit C	Thiamin B1	Riboflavin B2	Niacin B3	Iron	Calcium
Breakfast											
Snack											
Lunch											
Snack											
Dinner											
Snack											
Totals											

Food Consumed Today

Breakfast____

____

Snack____

____

Lunch____

____

____

Snack____
Dinner____

____

____

____

Snack____

Before starting any exercise program discuss it with your doctor or medical professional.

Fitness Journal
My Goals, My Training, and My Success

Motivation for eating healthy:_______________________
____
____
____

Immediate nutritional goals:________________________
____
____
____

Did I meet my nutritional goals today?________________
____
____

Long term nutritional or health related goals:_________
____
____
____

What changes in nutrition are necessary?
Increase Fluid Intake / Increase Fiber Intake / Decrease Unhealthy Foods /
Decrease Unhealthy Beverages / Increase Fruits or Vegetables / Increase Vitamin
or Mineral____
____
____
____

**Recent advice from doctor or other medical professional
regarding nutrition:**___________________________________
____
____

**Was it difficult to follow the nutritional advice from my
doctor or medical professional?**_______________________
____

Fitness Journal
My Goals, My Training, and My Success

My thoughts:

My Goals, My Training, and My Success

Fitness Journal 37

My Goals, My Training, and My Success

Name_________________________**Age**________**Date**__________

Fitness Trainer or Workout Partner_______________________________
Weight________Percent Body Fat________Blood Pressure__________
Resting Heart Rate___________Target Heart Rate________________
Medications____
____
Medical Problems____
____

Current Fitness Level
Never Exercise / Exercise Occasionally / Weekend Athlete / Exercise
Often / Competitive Athlete / High Fitness Level

____

____

What motivated me to begin a steady exercise program?
Doctor / Health Issues / Upcoming Event / Stress / Social Reasons

____

____

____

Long Term Fitness Goals
Weight Loss / Sculpt Body / Strength / Sports Specific / Health

____

____

____

3 Month Fitness Goals

____

____

____

1 Month Fitness Goals

____

____

____

I plan to exercise ________ days each week.

____

Before starting any exercise program discuss it with your doctor or medical professional.

My Goals, My Training, and My Success

How am I going to avoid distraction during workout today?

Goal for Today's Workout
Cardiovascular / Weight or Repetitions / Focus / Exercise Form / Other

What did I eat and drink before today's workout?

How do I feel before today's workout?
Energized / Motivated / Content / Drained / Exhausted / Unmotivated

Before starting any exercise program discuss it with your doctor or medical professional.

Fitness Journal
My Goals, My Training, and My Success

Strength Exercise Chart		
	Resistance	
	Repetitions	
	Sets	
	Resistance	
	Repetitions	
	Sets	
	Resistance	
	Repetitions	
	Sets	
	Resistance	
	Repetitions	
	Sets	
	Resistance	
	Repetitions	
	Sets	
	Resistance	
	Repetitions	
	Sets	
	Resistance	
	Repetitions	
	Sets	
	Resistance	
	Repetitions	
	Sets	
	Resistance	
	Repetitions	
	Sets	
Cardiovascular Exercise		
	Time	
	Time	
Stretching Exercise		
	Hold Time	
	Hold Time	
	Hold Time	
	Hold Time	

Before starting any exercise program discuss it with your doctor or medical professional.

Fitness Journal
My Goals, My Training, and My Success

Did I reach my goal for today?___________________________

____

____

How do I feel at end of today's workout?
Energized / Motivated / Content / Drained / Exhausted / Disappointed

____

____

____

Goals for next workout:_________________________________

____

____

____

Fitness Trainer's suggestions for next workout:________

____

____

____

Most recent advice from Health Care Professional
Health Status / Goals / Fitness Commitment

____

____

____

____

Were there any injuries or illnesses before or during today's workout?________________________________

____

____

____

My Goals, My Training, and My Success

Nutritional Section

A great way to discover whether you are getting all of the nutrients your body needs is to write down everything you eat for one week. Once you have the list compare the nutrient values in the foods you have consumed to the nutrient values recommended by your doctor or the recommended dietary allowance. Discuss the results with your doctor or other medical professional in order to improve or maintain your health.

Many people use a chart system similar to this one.

Food	Protein	Vit A	Vit D	Vit E	Vit K	Vit C	Thiamin B1	Riboflavin B2	Niacin B3	Iron	Calcium
Breakfast											
Snack											
Lunch											
Snack											
Dinner											
Snack											
Totals											

Food Consumed Today

Breakfast____

____

Snack____

____

Lunch____

____

____

____

Snack____
Dinner____

____

____

____

Snack____

Before starting any exercise program discuss it with your doctor or medical professional.

My Goals, My Training, and My Success

Motivation for eating healthy:_______________________

____

____

____

Immediate nutritional goals:________________________

____

____

____

Did I meet my nutritional goals today?________________

____

____

Long term nutritional or health related goals:__________

____

____

____

What changes in nutrition are necessary?
Increase Fluid Intake / Increase Fiber Intake / Decrease Unhealthy Foods /
Decrease Unhealthy Beverages / Increase Fruits or Vegetables / Increase Vitamin
or Mineral____

____

____

____

**Recent advice from doctor or other medical professional
regarding nutrition:**__________________________________

____

____

**Was it difficult to follow the nutritional advice from my
doctor or medical professional?**_______________________

____

Before starting any exercise program discuss it with your doctor or medical professional.

My Goals, My Training, and My Success

My thoughts:_______________________________________

My Goals, My Training, and My Success

Fitness Journal 45
My Goals, My Training, and My Success

Name_________________________________**Age**________**Date**__________

Fitness Trainer or Workout Partner_________________________________
Weight________Percent Body Fat________Blood Pressure__________
Resting Heart Rate___________Target Heart Rate_________________
Medications____

Medical Problems____

Current Fitness Level
Never Exercise / Exercise Occasionally / Weekend Athlete / Exercise
Often / Competitive Athlete / High Fitness Level

____

____

What motivated me to begin a steady exercise program?
Doctor / Health Issues / Upcoming Event / Stress / Social Reasons

____

____

____

Long Term Fitness Goals
Weight Loss / Sculpt Body / Strength / Sports Specific / Health

____

____

____

3 Month Fitness Goals

____

____

____

1 Month Fitness Goals

____

____

____

I plan to exercise _______ days each week.

____

Before starting any exercise program discuss it with your doctor or medical professional.

My Goals, My Training, and My Success

How am I going to avoid distraction during workout today?

____

____

Goal for Today's Workout

Cardiovascular / Weight or Repetitions / Focus / Exercise Form / Other

____

____

____

____

What did I eat and drink before today's workout?

____

____

____

____

How do I feel before today's workout?

Energized / Motivated / Content / Drained / Exhausted / Unmotivated

____

____

My Goals, My Training, and My Success

Strength Exercise Chart	
	Resistance
	Repetitions
	Sets
	Resistance
	Repetitions
	Sets
	Resistance
	Repetitions
	Sets
	Resistance
	Repetitions
	Sets
	Resistance
	Repetitions
	Sets
	Resistance
	Repetitions
	Sets
	Resistance
	Repetitions
	Sets
	Resistance
	Repetitions
	Sets
	Resistance
	Repetitions
	Sets
Cardiovascular Exercise	
	Time
	Time
Stretching Exercise	
	Hold Time
	Hold Time
	Hold Time
	Hold Time

Before starting any exercise program discuss it with your doctor or medical professional.

Fitness Journal
My Goals, My Training, and My Success

Did I reach my goal for today?_______________________
____
____

How do I feel at end of today's workout?
Energized / Motivated / Content / Drained / Exhausted / Disappointed
____
____
____

Goals for next workout:_______________________
____
____
____

Fitness Trainer's suggestions for next workout:________
____
____
____

Most recent advice from Health Care Professional
Health Status / Goals / Fitness Commitment
____
____
____
____

Were there any injuries or illnesses before or during today's workout?_______________________
____
____
____

Before starting any exercise program discuss it with your doctor or medical professional.

My Goals, My Training, and My Success

Nutritional Section

A great way to discover whether you are getting all of the nutrients your body needs is to write down everything you eat for one week. Once you have the list compare the nutrient values in the foods you have consumed to the nutrient values recommended by your doctor or the recommended dietary allowance. Discuss the results with your doctor or other medical professional in order to improve or maintain your health.

Many people use a chart system similar to this one.

Food	Protein	Vit A	Vit D	Vit E	Vit K	Vit C	Thiamin B1	Riboflavin B2	Niacin B3	Iron	Calcium
Breakfast											
Snack											
Lunch											
Snack											
Dinner											
Snack											
Totals											

Food Consumed Today

Breakfast____

____

Snack____

____

Lunch____

____

____

Snack____
Dinner____

____

____

Snack____

Before starting any exercise program discuss it with your doctor or medical professional.

My Goals, My Training, and My Success

Motivation for eating healthy:________________________________

____

____

____

Immediate nutritional goals:________________________

____

____

____

Did I meet my nutritional goals today?________________

____

____

Long term nutritional or health related goals:________

____

____

____

What changes in nutrition are necessary?
Increase Fluid Intake / Increase Fiber Intake / Decrease Unhealthy Foods /
Decrease Unhealthy Beverages / Increase Fruits or Vegetables / Increase Vitamin
or Mineral____

____

____

____

**Recent advice from doctor or other medical professional
regarding nutrition:**________________________________

____

____

**Was it difficult to follow the nutritional advice from my
doctor or medical professional?**________________________

____

Before starting any exercise program discuss it with your doctor or medical professional.

Fitness Journal
My Goals, My Training, and My Success

My thoughts:

Fitness Journal
My Goals, My Training, and My Success

Fitness Journal
My Goals, My Training, and My Success

Name____________________________**Age**________**Date**__________

Fitness Trainer or Workout Partner___________________________
Weight________Percent Body Fat________Blood Pressure__________
Resting Heart Rate___________Target Heart Rate__________________
Medications____

Medical Problems____

Current Fitness Level
Never Exercise / Exercise Occasionally / Weekend Athlete / Exercise Often / Competitive Athlete / High Fitness Level

What motivated me to begin a steady exercise program?
Doctor / Health Issues / Upcoming Event / Stress / Social Reasons

Long Term Fitness Goals
Weight Loss / Sculpt Body / Strength / Sports Specific / Health

3 Month Fitness Goals

1 Month Fitness Goals

I plan to exercise _______ days each week.

Before starting any exercise program discuss it with your doctor or medical professional.

My Goals, My Training, and My Success

How am I going to avoid distraction during workout today?

____

____

Goal for Today's Workout
Cardiovascular / Weight or Repetitions / Focus / Exercise Form / Other

____

____

____

____

What did I eat and drink before today's workout?

____

____

____

____

How do I feel before today's workout?
Energized / Motivated / Content / Drained / Exhausted / Unmotivated

____

____

Fitness Journal
My Goals, My Training, and My Success

Strength Exercise Chart		
	Resistance	
	Repetitions	
	Sets	
	Resistance	
	Repetitions	
	Sets	
	Resistance	
	Repetitions	
	Sets	
	Resistance	
	Repetitions	
	Sets	
	Resistance	
	Repetitions	
	Sets	
	Resistance	
	Repetitions	
	Sets	
	Resistance	
	Repetitions	
	Sets	
	Resistance	
	Repetitions	
	Sets	
	Resistance	
	Repetitions	
	Sets	
Cardiovascular Exercise		
	Time	
	Time	
Stretching Exercise		
	Hold Time	
	Hold Time	
	Hold Time	
	Hold Time	

Before starting any exercise program discuss it with your doctor or medical professional.

Fitness Journal
My Goals, My Training, and My Success

Did I reach my goal for today?______________________

____
____

How do I feel at end of today's workout?
Energized / Motivated / Content / Drained / Exhausted / Disappointed

____
____
____

Goals for next workout:______________________

____
____
____

Fitness Trainer's suggestions for next workout:______

____
____
____

Most recent advice from Health Care Professional
Health Status / Goals / Fitness Commitment

____
____
____
____

Were there any injuries or illnesses before or during today's workout?______________________

____
____
____

Before starting any exercise program discuss it with your doctor or medical professional.

My Goals, My Training, and My Success

Nutritional Section

A great way to discover whether you are getting all of the nutrients your body needs is to write down everything you eat for one week. Once you have the list compare the nutrient values in the foods you have consumed to the nutrient values recommended by your doctor or the recommended dietary allowance. Discuss the results with your doctor or other medical professional in order to improve or maintain your health.

Many people use a chart system similar to this one.

Food	Protein	Vit A	Vit D	Vit E	Vit K	Vit C	Thiamin B1	Riboflavin B2	Niacin B3	Iron	Calcium
Breakfast											
Snack											
Lunch											
Snack											
Dinner											
Snack											
Totals											

Food Consumed Today

Breakfast____

____

Snack____

____

Lunch____

____

____

____

Snack____
Dinner____

____

____

____

Snack____

My Goals, My Training, and My Success

Motivation for eating healthy:_________________________

____

____

____

Immediate nutritional goals:_________________________

____

____

____

Did I meet my nutritional goals today?_________________

____

____

Long term nutritional or health related goals:__________

____

____

____

What changes in nutrition are necessary?
Increase Fluid Intake / Increase Fiber Intake / Decrease Unhealthy Foods /
Decrease Unhealthy Beverages / Increase Fruits or Vegetables / Increase Vitamin
or Mineral____

____

____

____

____

**Recent advice from doctor or other medical professional
regarding nutrition:**____________________________________

____

____

____

**Was it difficult to follow the nutritional advice from my
doctor or medical professional?**________________________

____

Before starting any exercise program discuss it with your doctor or medical professional.

Fitness Journal
My Goals, My Training, and My Success

My thoughts:

My Goals, My Training, and My Success

Fitness Journal 61

My Goals, My Training, and My Success

Name________________________________**Age**________**Date**__________

Fitness Trainer or Workout Partner________________________________
Weight________Percent Body Fat________Blood Pressure__________
Resting Heart Rate___________Target Heart Rate___________________
Medications____

____
Medical Problems____

____

Current Fitness Level
Never Exercise / Exercise Occasionally / Weekend Athlete / Exercise
Often / Competitive Athlete / High Fitness Level

____

____

What motivated me to begin a steady exercise program?
Doctor / Health Issues / Upcoming Event / Stress / Social Reasons

____

____

____

Long Term Fitness Goals
Weight Loss / Sculpt Body / Strength / Sports Specific / Health

____

____

____

3 Month Fitness Goals

____

____

____

1 Month Fitness Goals

____

____

____

I plan to exercise ________ days each week.

____

Before starting any exercise program discuss it with your doctor or medical professional.

My Goals, My Training, and My Success

How am I going to avoid distraction during workout today?

____

____

Goal for Today's Workout
Cardiovascular / Weight or Repetitions / Focus / Exercise Form / Other

____

____

____

____

What did I eat and drink before today's workout?

____

____

____

____

How do I feel before today's workout?
Energized / Motivated / Content / Drained / Exhausted / Unmotivated

____

____

My Goals, My Training, and My Success

Strength Exercise Chart		
	Resistance	
	Repetitions	
	Sets	
	Resistance	
	Repetitions	
	Sets	
	Resistance	
	Repetitions	
	Sets	
	Resistance	
	Repetitions	
	Sets	
	Resistance	
	Repetitions	
	Sets	
	Resistance	
	Repetitions	
	Sets	
	Resistance	
	Repetitions	
	Sets	
	Resistance	
	Repetitions	
	Sets	
	Resistance	
	Repetitions	
	Sets	
Cardiovascular Exercise		
	Time	
	Time	
Stretching Exercise		
	Hold Time	
	Hold Time	
	Hold Time	
	Hold Time	

Before starting any exercise program discuss it with your doctor or medical professional.

Fitness Journal
My Goals, My Training, and My Success

Did I reach my goal for today?________________________

____

____

How do I feel at end of today's workout?
Energized / Motivated / Content / Drained / Exhausted / Disappointed

____

____

____

Goals for next workout:________________________________

____

____

____

Fitness Trainer's suggestions for next workout:________

____

____

____

Most recent advice from Health Care Professional
Health Status / Goals / Fitness Commitment

____

____

____

____

Were there any injuries or illnesses before or during today's workout?_______________________________________

____

____

____

Fitness Journal
My Goals, My Training, and My Success

Nutritional Section

A great way to discover whether you are getting all of the nutrients your body needs is to write down everything you eat for one week. Once you have the list compare the nutrient values in the foods you have consumed to the nutrient values recommended by your doctor or the recommended dietary allowance. Discuss the results with your doctor or other medical professional in order to improve or maintain your health.

Many people use a chart system similar to this one.

Food	Protein	Vit A	Vit D	Vit E	Vit K	Vit C	Thiamin B1	Riboflavin B2	Niacin B3	Iron	Calcium
Breakfast											
Snack											
Lunch											
Snack											
Dinner											
Snack											
Totals											

Food Consumed Today

Breakfast____

____

Snack____

____

Lunch____

____

____

Snack____
Dinner____

____

____

Snack____

Before starting any exercise program discuss it with your doctor or medical professional.

My Goals, My Training, and My Success

Motivation for eating healthy:_______________________

____

____

____

Immediate nutritional goals:_________________________

____

____

____

Did I meet my nutritional goals today?_______________

____

____

Long term nutritional or health related goals:_________

____

____

____

What changes in nutrition are necessary?

Increase Fluid Intake / Increase Fiber Intake / Decrease Unhealthy Foods / Decrease Unhealthy Beverages / Increase Fruits or Vegetables / Increase Vitamin or Mineral_______________________________________

____

____

____

____

Recent advice from doctor or other medical professional regarding nutrition:_________________________________

____

____

____

Was it difficult to follow the nutritional advice from my doctor or medical professional?_______________________

____

Fitness Journal
My Goals, My Training, and My Success

My thoughts:

Fitness Journal

My Goals, My Training, and My Success

Before starting any exercise program discuss it with your doctor or medical professional.

Fitness Journal

My Goals, My Training, and My Success

Name________________________________**Age**_________**Date**___________

Fitness Trainer or Workout Partner__________________________________
Weight_________Percent Body Fat_________Blood Pressure___________
Resting Heart Rate_____________Target Heart Rate______________________
Medications____

Medical Problems____

Current Fitness Level
Never Exercise / Exercise Occasionally / Weekend Athlete / Exercise
Often / Competitive Athlete / High Fitness Level

What motivated me to begin a steady exercise program?
Doctor / Health Issues / Upcoming Event / Stress / Social Reasons

Long Term Fitness Goals
Weight Loss / Sculpt Body / Strength / Sports Specific / Health

3 Month Fitness Goals

1 Month Fitness Goals

I plan to exercise _______ days each week.

Before starting any exercise program discuss it with your doctor or medical professional.

My Goals, My Training, and My Success

How am I going to avoid distraction during workout today?

____

____

Goal for Today's Workout
Cardiovascular / Weight or Repetitions / Focus / Exercise Form / Other

____

____

____

____

What did I eat and drink before today's workout?

____

____

____

____

How do I feel before today's workout?
Energized / Motivated / Content / Drained / Exhausted / Unmotivated

____

____

Fitness Journal
My Goals, My Training, and My Success

Strength Exercise Chart	
	Resistance
	Repetitions
	Sets
	Resistance
	Repetitions
	Sets
	Resistance
	Repetitions
	Sets
	Resistance
	Repetitions
	Sets
	Resistance
	Repetitions
	Sets
	Resistance
	Repetitions
	Sets
	Resistance
	Repetitions
	Sets
	Resistance
	Repetitions
	Sets
	Resistance
	Repetitions
	Sets
Cardiovascular Exercise	
	Time
	Time
Stretching Exercise	
	Hold Time
	Hold Time
	Hold Time
	Hold Time

Before starting any exercise program discuss it with your doctor or medical professional.

Fitness Journal
My Goals, My Training, and My Success

Did I reach my goal for today?______________________

____

____

How do I feel at end of today's workout?
Energized / Motivated / Content / Drained / Exhausted / Disappointed

____

____

____

Goals for next workout:______________________

____

____

____

Fitness Trainer's suggestions for next workout:______

____

____

____

Most recent advice from Health Care Professional
Health Status / Goals / Fitness Commitment

____

____

____

____

Were there any injuries or illnesses before or during today's workout?______________________

____

____

____

My Goals, My Training, and My Success

Nutritional Section

A great way to discover whether you are getting all of the nutrients your body needs is to write down everything you eat for one week. Once you have the list compare the nutrient values in the foods you have consumed to the nutrient values recommended by your doctor or the recommended dietary allowance. Discuss the results with your doctor or other medical professional in order to improve or maintain your health.

Many people use a chart system similar to this one.

Food	Protein	Vit A	Vit D	Vit E	Vit K	Vit C	Thiamin B1	Riboflavin B2	Niacin B3	Iron	Calcium
Breakfast											
Snack											
Lunch											
Snack											
Dinner											
Snack											
Totals											

Food Consumed Today

Breakfast____

____

Snack____

____

Lunch____

____

____

Snack____
Dinner____

____

____

Snack____

Fitness Journal
My Goals, My Training, and My Success

Motivation for eating healthy:________________________

____
____
____

Immediate nutritional goals:__________________________

____
____
____

Did I meet my nutritional goals today?_______________

____
____

Long term nutritional or health related goals:_________

____
____
____

What changes in nutrition are necessary?
Increase Fluid Intake / Increase Fiber Intake / Decrease Unhealthy Foods /
Decrease Unhealthy Beverages / Increase Fruits or Vegetables / Increase Vitamin
or Mineral_______________________________________

____
____
____
____

**Recent advice from doctor or other medical professional
regarding nutrition:**___________________________

____
____
____

**Was it difficult to follow the nutritional advice from my
doctor or medical professional?**__________________

____

Fitness Journal
My Goals, My Training, and My Success

My thoughts:

Fitness Journal

My Goals, My Training, and My Success

Fitness Journal

My Goals, My Training, and My Success

Name_______________________________**Age**________**Date**__________

Fitness Trainer or Workout Partner_________________________________
Weight________Percent Body Fat________Blood Pressure__________
Resting Heart Rate___________Target Heart Rate__________________
Medications____

____
Medical Problems____

____

Current Fitness Level
Never Exercise / Exercise Occasionally / Weekend Athlete / Exercise
Often / Competitive Athlete / High Fitness Level

____

____

What motivated me to begin a steady exercise program?
Doctor / Health Issues / Upcoming Event / Stress / Social Reasons

____

____

____

Long Term Fitness Goals
Weight Loss / Sculpt Body / Strength / Sports Specific / Health

____

____

____

3 Month Fitness Goals

____

____

____

1 Month Fitness Goals

____

____

____

I plan to exercise _______ days each week.

____

Before starting any exercise program discuss it with your doctor or medical professional.

Fitness Journal
My Goals, My Training, and My Success

How am I going to avoid distraction during workout today?

Goal for Today's Workout
Cardiovascular / Weight or Repetitions / Focus / Exercise Form / Other

---

What did I eat and drink before today's workout?

How do I feel before today's workout?
Energized / Motivated / Content / Drained / Exhausted / Unmotivated

---

Fitness Journal
My Goals, My Training, and My Success

Strength Exercise Chart		
	Resistance	
	Repetitions	
	Sets	
	Resistance	
	Repetitions	
	Sets	
	Resistance	
	Repetitions	
	Sets	
	Resistance	
	Repetitions	
	Sets	
	Resistance	
	Repetitions	
	Sets	
	Resistance	
	Repetitions	
	Sets	
	Resistance	
	Repetitions	
	Sets	
	Resistance	
	Repetitions	
	Sets	
Cardiovascular Exercise		
	Time	
	Time	
Stretching Exercise		
	Hold Time	
	Hold Time	
	Hold Time	
	Hold Time	

Before starting any exercise program discuss it with your doctor or medical professional.

Fitness Journal
My Goals, My Training, and My Success

Did I reach my goal for today?_______________________
____
____

How do I feel at end of today's workout?
Energized / Motivated / Content / Drained / Exhausted / Disappointed

____
____
____

Goals for next workout:_________________________________
____
____
____

Fitness Trainer's suggestions for next workout:________
____
____
____

Most recent advice from Health Care Professional
Health Status / Goals / Fitness Commitment

____
____
____
____

Were there any injuries or illnesses before or during today's workout?____
____
____
____

My Goals, My Training, and My Success

Nutritional Section

A great way to discover whether you are getting all of the nutrients your body needs is to write down everything you eat for one week. Once you have the list compare the nutrient values in the foods you have consumed to the nutrient values recommended by your doctor or the recommended dietary allowance. Discuss the results with your doctor or other medical professional in order to improve or maintain your health.

Many people use a chart system similar to this one.

Food	Protein	Vit A	Vit D	Vit E	Vit K	Vit C	Thiamin B1	Riboflavin B2	Niacin B3	Iron	Calcium
Breakfast											
Snack											
Lunch											
Snack											
Dinner											
Snack											
Totals											

Food Consumed Today

Breakfast____

____

Snack____

____

Lunch____

____

____

Snack____
Dinner____

____

____

Snack____

Before starting any exercise program discuss it with your doctor or medical professional.

Fitness Journal
My Goals, My Training, and My Success

Motivation for eating healthy:______________________________
____
____
____

Immediate nutritional goals:________________________________
____
____
____

Did I meet my nutritional goals today?__________________
____
____

Long term nutritional or health related goals:__________
____
____
____

What changes in nutrition are necessary?
Increase Fluid Intake / Increase Fiber Intake / Decrease Unhealthy Foods /
Decrease Unhealthy Beverages / Increase Fruits or Vegetables / Increase Vitamin
or Mineral____
____
____
____
____

Recent advice from doctor or other medical professional regarding nutrition:__________________________________
____
____
____

Was it difficult to follow the nutritional advice from my doctor or medical professional?___________________
____

Fitness Journal
My Goals, My Training, and My Success

My thoughts:

Before starting any exercise program discuss it with your doctor or medical professional.

Fitness Journal
My Goals, My Training, and My Success

Fitness Journal
My Goals, My Training, and My Success

Name_____________________________**Age**________**Date**__________

Fitness Trainer or Workout Partner_________________________________
Weight__________Percent Body Fat_________Blood Pressure___________
Resting Heart Rate_____________Target Heart Rate_________________
Medications____
____
Medical Problems____
____

Current Fitness Level
Never Exercise / Exercise Occasionally / Weekend Athlete / Exercise
Often / Competitive Athlete / High Fitness Level

____
____

What motivated me to begin a steady exercise program?
Doctor / Health Issues / Upcoming Event / Stress / Social Reasons

____
____
____

Long Term Fitness Goals
Weight Loss / Sculpt Body / Strength / Sports Specific / Health

____
____
____

3 Month Fitness Goals

____
____
____

1 Month Fitness Goals

____
____
____

I plan to exercise _______ days each week.

____

Before starting any exercise program discuss it with your doctor or medical professional.

My Goals, My Training, and My Success

How am I going to avoid distraction during workout today?

____

____

Goal for Today's Workout
Cardiovascular / Weight or Repetitions / Focus / Exercise Form / Other

____

____

____

____

What did I eat and drink before today's workout?

____

____

____

____

How do I feel before today's workout?
Energized / Motivated / Content / Drained / Exhausted / Unmotivated

____

____

My Goals, My Training, and My Success

Strength Exercise Chart	
	Resistance
	Repetitions
	Sets
	Resistance
	Repetitions
	Sets
	Resistance
	Repetitions
	Sets
	Resistance
	Repetitions
	Sets
	Resistance
	Repetitions
	Sets
	Resistance
	Repetitions
	Sets
	Resistance
	Repetitions
	Sets
	Resistance
	Repetitions
	Sets
	Resistance
	Repetitions
	Sets
Cardiovascular Exercise	
	Time
	Time
Stretching Exercise	
	Hold Time
	Hold Time
	Hold Time
	Hold Time

Before starting any exercise program discuss it with your doctor or medical professional.

Fitness Journal
My Goals, My Training, and My Success

Did I reach my goal for today?

How do I feel at end of today's workout?
Energized / Motivated / Content / Drained / Exhausted / Disappointed

Goals for next workout:

Fitness Trainer's suggestions for next workout:

Most recent advice from Health Care Professional
Health Status / Goals / Fitness Commitment

Were there any injuries or illnesses before or during today's workout?

My Goals, My Training, and My Success

Nutritional Section

A great way to discover whether you are getting all of the nutrients your body needs is to write down everything you eat for one week. Once you have the list compare the nutrient values in the foods you have consumed to the nutrient values recommended by your doctor or the recommended dietary allowance. Discuss the results with your doctor or other medical professional in order to improve or maintain your health.

Many people use a chart system similar to this one.

Food	Protein	Vit A	Vit D	Vit E	Vit K	Vit C	Thiamin B1	Riboflavin B2	Niacin B3	Iron	Calcium
Breakfast											
Snack											
Lunch											
Snack											
Dinner											
Snack											
Totals											

Food Consumed Today

Breakfast____

____

Snack____

____

Lunch____

____

____

Snack____
Dinner____

____

____

Snack____

Before starting any exercise program discuss it with your doctor or medical professional.

My Goals, My Training, and My Success

Motivation for eating healthy:_______________________
____
____
____

Immediate nutritional goals:_______________________
____
____
____

Did I meet my nutritional goals today?_______________
____
____

Long term nutritional or health related goals:__________
____
____
____

What changes in nutrition are necessary?
Increase Fluid Intake / Increase Fiber Intake / Decrease Unhealthy Foods /
Decrease Unhealthy Beverages / Increase Fruits or Vegetables / Increase Vitamin
or Mineral_______________________________________
____
____
____

**Recent advice from doctor or other medical professional
regarding nutrition:**___________________________
____
____

**Was it difficult to follow the nutritional advice from my
doctor or medical professional?**____________________
____

Before starting any exercise program discuss it with your doctor or medical professional.

Fitness Journal
My Goals, My Training, and My Success

My thoughts:

Fitness Journal
My Goals, My Training, and My Success

Fitness Journal 93
My Goals, My Training, and My Success

Name___________________________**Age**________**Date**__________

Fitness Trainer or Workout Partner______________________________
Weight________Percent Body Fat________Blood Pressure__________
Resting Heart Rate___________Target Heart Rate_________________
Medications____
____
Medical Problems____
____

Current Fitness Level
Never Exercise / Exercise Occasionally / Weekend Athlete / Exercise Often / Competitive Athlete / High Fitness Level

____

____

What motivated me to begin a steady exercise program?
Doctor / Health Issues / Upcoming Event / Stress / Social Reasons

____

____

____

Long Term Fitness Goals
Weight Loss / Sculpt Body / Strength / Sports Specific / Health

____

____

____

3 Month Fitness Goals

____

____

____

1 Month Fitness Goals

____

____

____

I plan to exercise _______ days each week.

____

Before starting any exercise program discuss it with your doctor or medical professional.

Fitness Journal
My Goals, My Training, and My Success

How am I going to avoid distraction during workout today?

____

____

Goal for Today's Workout
Cardiovascular / Weight or Repetitions / Focus / Exercise Form / Other

____

____

____

____

What did I eat and drink before today's workout?

____

____

____

____

How do I feel before today's workout?
Energized / Motivated / Content / Drained / Exhausted / Unmotivated

____

____

Fitness Journal
My Goals, My Training, and My Success

Strength Exercise Chart	
	Resistance
	Repetitions
	Sets
	Resistance
	Repetitions
	Sets
	Resistance
	Repetitions
	Sets
	Resistance
	Repetitions
	Sets
	Resistance
	Repetitions
	Sets
	Resistance
	Repetitions
	Sets
	Resistance
	Repetitions
	Sets
	Resistance
	Repetitions
	Sets
	Resistance
	Repetitions
	Sets
Cardiovascular Exercise	
	Time
	Time
Stretching Exercise	
	Hold Time
	Hold Time
	Hold Time
	Hold Time

Before starting any exercise program discuss it with your doctor or medical professional.

Fitness Journal
My Goals, My Training, and My Success

Did I reach my goal for today?______________________
____
____

How do I feel at end of today's workout?
Energized / Motivated / Content / Drained / Exhausted / Disappointed
____
____
____

Goals for next workout:______________________
____
____
____

Fitness Trainer's suggestions for next workout:______
____
____
____

Most recent advice from Health Care Professional
Health Status / Goals / Fitness Commitment
____
____
____
____

Were there any injuries or illnesses before or during today's workout?______________________
____
____
____

My Goals, My Training, and My Success

Nutritional Section

A great way to discover whether you are getting all of the nutrients your body needs is to write down everything you eat for one week. Once you have the list compare the nutrient values in the foods you have consumed to the nutrient values recommended by your doctor or the recommended dietary allowance. Discuss the results with your doctor or other medical professional in order to improve or maintain your health.

Many people use a chart system similar to this one.

Food	Protein	Vit A	Vit D	Vit E	Vit K	Vit C	Thiamin B1	Riboflavin B2	Niacin B3	Iron	Calcium
Breakfast											
Snack											
Lunch											
Snack											
Dinner											
Snack											
Totals											

Food Consumed Today

Breakfast____

____

Snack____

____

Lunch____

____

____

Snack____
Dinner____

____

____

Snack____

Before starting any exercise program discuss it with your doctor or medical professional.

My Goals, My Training, and My Success

Motivation for eating healthy:___________________________

____

____

____

Immediate nutritional goals:____________________________

____

____

____

Did I meet my nutritional goals today?___________________

____

____

Long term nutritional or health related goals:__________

____

____

____

What changes in nutrition are necessary?
Increase Fluid Intake / Increase Fiber Intake / Decrease Unhealthy Foods /
Decrease Unhealthy Beverages / Increase Fruits or Vegetables / Increase Vitamin
or Mineral____

____

____

____

____

**Recent advice from doctor or other medical professional
regarding nutrition:**_____________________________________

____

____

____

**Was it difficult to follow the nutritional advice from my
doctor or medical professional?**__________________________

____

My Goals, My Training, and My Success

My thoughts:_______________________________

Fitness Journal
My Goals, My Training, and My Success

Fitness Journal
My Goals, My Training, and My Success

Name___________________________**Age**_________**Date**___________

Fitness Trainer or Workout Partner_______________________________
Weight__________Percent Body Fat_________Blood Pressure___________
Resting Heart Rate_____________Target Heart Rate__________________
Medications____
____
Medical Problems____
____

Current Fitness Level
Never Exercise / Exercise Occasionally / Weekend Athlete / Exercise
Often / Competitive Athlete / High Fitness Level

____

____

What motivated me to begin a steady exercise program?
Doctor / Health Issues / Upcoming Event / Stress / Social Reasons

____

____

____

Long Term Fitness Goals
Weight Loss / Sculpt Body / Strength / Sports Specific / Health

____

____

____

3 Month Fitness Goals

____

____

____

1 Month Fitness Goals

____

____

____

I plan to exercise _______ days each week.

____

Before starting any exercise program discuss it with your doctor or medical professional.

My Goals, My Training, and My Success

How am I going to avoid distraction during workout today?

____

____

Goal for Today's Workout
Cardiovascular / Weight or Repetitions / Focus / Exercise Form / Other

____

____

____

____

What did I eat and drink before today's workout?

____

____

____

____

How do I feel before today's workout?
Energized / Motivated / Content / Drained / Exhausted / Unmotivated

____

____

Fitness Journal
My Goals, My Training, and My Success

Strength Exercise Chart		
	Resistance	
	Repetitions	
	Sets	
	Resistance	
	Repetitions	
	Sets	
	Resistance	
	Repetitions	
	Sets	
	Resistance	
	Repetitions	
	Sets	
	Resistance	
	Repetitions	
	Sets	
	Resistance	
	Repetitions	
	Sets	
	Resistance	
	Repetitions	
	Sets	
	Resistance	
	Repetitions	
	Sets	
	Resistance	
	Repetitions	
	Sets	
Cardiovascular Exercise		
	Time	
	Time	
Stretching Exercise		
	Hold Time	
	Hold Time	
	Hold Time	
	Hold Time	

Before starting any exercise program discuss it with your doctor or medical professional.

Fitness Journal
My Goals, My Training, and My Success

Did I reach my goal for today?________________________
____
____

How do I feel at end of today's workout?
Energized / Motivated / Content / Drained / Exhausted / Disappointed
____
____
____

Goals for next workout:________________________________
____
____
____

Fitness Trainer's suggestions for next workout:________
____
____
____

Most recent advice from Health Care Professional
Health Status / Goals / Fitness Commitment
____
____
____
____

Were there any injuries or illnesses before or during today's workout?________________________________
____
____
____

My Goals, My Training, and My Success

Nutritional Section

A great way to discover whether you are getting all of the nutrients your body needs is to write down everything you eat for one week. Once you have the list compare the nutrient values in the foods you have consumed to the nutrient values recommended by your doctor or the recommended dietary allowance. Discuss the results with your doctor or other medical professional in order to improve or maintain your health.

Many people use a chart system similar to this one.

Food	Protein	Vit A	Vit D	Vit E	Vit K	Vit C	Thiamin B1	Riboflavin B2	Niacin B3	Iron	Calcium
Breakfast											
Snack											
Lunch											
Snack											
Dinner											
Snack											
Totals											

Food Consumed Today

Breakfast____

____

Snack____

____

Lunch____

____

____

Snack____

Dinner____

____

____

Snack____

Before starting any exercise program discuss it with your doctor or medical professional.

My Goals, My Training, and My Success

Motivation for eating healthy:_______________________

____

____

____

Immediate nutritional goals:________________________

____

____

____

Did I meet my nutritional goals today?________________

____

____

Long term nutritional or health related goals:__________

____

____

____

What changes in nutrition are necessary?
Increase Fluid Intake / Increase Fiber Intake / Decrease Unhealthy Foods / Decrease Unhealthy Beverages / Increase Fruits or Vegetables / Increase Vitamin or Mineral_______________________________________

____

____

____

____

Recent advice from doctor or other medical professional regarding nutrition:______________________________

____

____

____

Was it difficult to follow the nutritional advice from my doctor or medical professional?___________________

____

My Goals, My Training, and My Success

My thoughts:

My Goals, My Training, and My Success

Fitness Journal
My Goals, My Training, and My Success

Name_______________________________**Age**__________**Date**___________

Fitness Trainer or Workout Partner_____________________________
Weight__________Percent Body Fat__________Blood Pressure___________
Resting Heart Rate_____________Target Heart Rate_____________________
Medications____
____
Medical Problems____
____

Current Fitness Level
Never Exercise / Exercise Occasionally / Weekend Athlete / Exercise
Often / Competitive Athlete / High Fitness Level

____

____

What motivated me to begin a steady exercise program?
Doctor / Health Issues / Upcoming Event / Stress / Social Reasons

____

____

____

Long Term Fitness Goals
Weight Loss / Sculpt Body / Strength / Sports Specific / Health

____

____

____

3 Month Fitness Goals

____

____

____

1 Month Fitness Goals

____

____

____

I plan to exercise _________ days each week.

____

Before starting any exercise program discuss it with your doctor or medical professional.

How am I going to avoid distraction during workout today?

____

____

Goal for Today's Workout

Cardiovascular / Weight or Repetitions / Focus / Exercise Form / Other

____

____

____

____

What did I eat and drink before today's workout?

____

____

____

____

How do I feel before today's workout?

Energized / Motivated / Content / Drained / Exhausted / Unmotivated

____

____

My Goals, My Training, and My Success

Strength Exercise Chart	
	Resistance
	Repetitions
	Sets
	Resistance
	Repetitions
	Sets
	Resistance
	Repetitions
	Sets
	Resistance
	Repetitions
	Sets
	Resistance
	Repetitions
	Sets
	Resistance
	Repetitions
	Sets
	Resistance
	Repetitions
	Sets
	Resistance
	Repetitions
	Sets
	Resistance
	Repetitions
	Sets
Cardiovascular Exercise	
	Time
	Time
Stretching Exercise	
	Hold Time
	Hold Time
	Hold Time
	Hold Time

Before starting any exercise program discuss it with your doctor or medical professional.

Fitness Journal
My Goals, My Training, and My Success

Did I reach my goal for today?___________________

____

____

How do I feel at end of today's workout?
Energized / Motivated / Content / Drained / Exhausted / Disappointed

____

____

____

Goals for next workout:___________________________

____

____

____

Fitness Trainer's suggestions for next workout:________

____

____

____

Most recent advice from Health Care Professional
Health Status / Goals / Fitness Commitment

____

____

____

____

Were there any injuries or illnesses before or during today's workout?___________________________________

____

____

____

Fitness Journal
My Goals, My Training, and My Success

Nutritional Section

A great way to discover whether you are getting all of the nutrients your body needs is to write down everything you eat for one week. Once you have the list compare the nutrient values in the foods you have consumed to the nutrient values recommended by your doctor or the recommended dietary allowance. Discuss the results with your doctor or other medical professional in order to improve or maintain your health.

Many people use a chart system similar to this one.

Food	Protein	Vit A	Vit D	Vit E	Vit K	Vit C	Thiamin B1	Riboflavin B2	Niacin B3	Iron	Calcium
Breakfast											
Snack											
Lunch											
Snack											
Dinner											
Snack											
Totals											

Food Consumed Today

Breakfast____

____

Snack____

____

Lunch____

____

____

Snack____
Dinner____

____

____

____

Snack____

My Goals, My Training, and My Success

Motivation for eating healthy:______________________

____

____

____

Immediate nutritional goals:______________________

____

____

____

Did I meet my nutritional goals today?______________

____

____

Long term nutritional or health related goals:________

____

____

____

What changes in nutrition are necessary?
Increase Fluid Intake / Increase Fiber Intake / Decrease Unhealthy Foods /
Decrease Unhealthy Beverages / Increase Fruits or Vegetables / Increase Vitamin
or Mineral______________________

____

____

____

____

**Recent advice from doctor or other medical professional
regarding nutrition:**______________________

____

____

____

**Was it difficult to follow the nutritional advice from my
doctor or medical professional?**______________________

____

Before starting any exercise program discuss it with your doctor or medical professional.

My Goals, My Training, and My Success

My thoughts:

Fitness Journal
My Goals, My Training, and My Success

Fitness Journal
My Goals, My Training, and My Success

Name___________________________**Age**________**Date**__________

Fitness Trainer or Workout Partner___________________________________
Weight_________Percent Body Fat_________Blood Pressure___________
Resting Heart Rate____________Target Heart Rate_______________________
Medications____
____
Medical Problems____
____

Current Fitness Level
Never Exercise / Exercise Occasionally / Weekend Athlete / Exercise Often / Competitive Athlete / High Fitness Level

____

____

What motivated me to begin a steady exercise program?
Doctor / Health Issues / Upcoming Event / Stress / Social Reasons

____

____

____

Long Term Fitness Goals
Weight Loss / Sculpt Body / Strength / Sports Specific / Health

____

____

____

3 Month Fitness Goals

____

____

____

1 Month Fitness Goals

____

____

____

I plan to exercise _______ days each week.

____

Before starting any exercise program discuss it with your doctor or medical professional.

My Goals, My Training, and My Success

How am I going to avoid distraction during workout today?

____

____

Goal for Today's Workout
Cardiovascular / Weight or Repetitions / Focus / Exercise Form / Other

____

____

____

____

What did I eat and drink before today's workout?

____

____

____

____

How do I feel before today's workout?
Energized / Motivated / Content / Drained / Exhausted / Unmotivated

____

____

My Goals, My Training, and My Success

Strength Exercise Chart	
	Resistance
	Repetitions
	Sets
	Resistance
	Repetitions
	Sets
	Resistance
	Repetitions
	Sets
	Resistance
	Repetitions
	Sets
	Resistance
	Repetitions
	Sets
	Resistance
	Repetitions
	Sets
	Resistance
	Repetitions
	Sets
	Resistance
	Repetitions
	Sets
	Resistance
	Repetitions
	Sets
Cardiovascular Exercise	
	Time
	Time
Stretching Exercise	
	Hold Time
	Hold Time
	Hold Time
	Hold Time

Before starting any exercise program discuss it with your doctor or medical professional.

Fitness Journal
My Goals, My Training, and My Success

Did I reach my goal for today?_____________________

____

____

How do I feel at end of today's workout?
Energized / Motivated / Content / Drained / Exhausted / Disappointed

____

____

____

Goals for next workout:_____________________________

____

____

____

Fitness Trainer's suggestions for next workout:________

____

____

____

Most recent advice from Health Care Professional
Health Status / Goals / Fitness Commitment

____

____

____

____

Were there any injuries or illnesses before or during today's workout?___________________________________

____

____

____

Nutritional Section

A great way to discover whether you are getting all of the nutrients your body needs is to write down everything you eat for one week. Once you have the list compare the nutrient values in the foods you have consumed to the nutrient values recommended by your doctor or the recommended dietary allowance. Discuss the results with your doctor or other medical professional in order to improve or maintain your health.

Many people use a chart system similar to this one.

Food	Protein	Vit A	Vit D	Vit E	Vit K	Vit C	Thiamin B1	Riboflavin B2	Niacin B3	Iron	Calcium
Breakfast											
Snack											
Lunch											
Snack											
Dinner											
Snack											
Totals											

Food Consumed Today

Breakfast____

____

Snack____

____

Lunch____

____

____

Snack____
Dinner____

____

____

Snack____

Before starting any exercise program discuss it with your doctor or medical professional.

My Goals, My Training, and My Success

Motivation for eating healthy:_______________________

____
____
____

Immediate nutritional goals:_______________________

____
____
____

Did I meet my nutritional goals today?_______________

____
____

Long term nutritional or health related goals:________

____
____
____

What changes in nutrition are necessary?
Increase Fluid Intake / Increase Fiber Intake / Decrease Unhealthy Foods /
Decrease Unhealthy Beverages / Increase Fruits or Vegetables / Increase Vitamin
or Mineral____

____
____
____
____

**Recent advice from doctor or other medical professional
regarding nutrition:**___________________________________

____
____
____

**Was it difficult to follow the nutritional advice from my
doctor or medical professional?**________________________

____

Before starting any exercise program discuss it with your doctor or medical professional.

My Goals, My Training, and My Success

My thoughts:____

____

____

____

____

____

____

____

____

____

____

____

____

____

____

____

____

____

____

____

____

____

____

____

____

____

____

____

____

____

Fitness Journal
My Goals, My Training, and My Success

Fitness Journal
My Goals, My Training, and My Success

Name___________________________________**Age**_________**Date**__________

Fitness Trainer or Workout Partner_____________________________________
Weight_________Percent Body Fat_________Blood Pressure___________
Resting Heart Rate_____________Target Heart Rate_______________________
Medications____

Medical Problems____

Current Fitness Level
Never Exercise / Exercise Occasionally / Weekend Athlete / Exercise
Often / Competitive Athlete / High Fitness Level

What motivated me to begin a steady exercise program?
Doctor / Health Issues / Upcoming Event / Stress / Social Reasons

Long Term Fitness Goals
Weight Loss / Sculpt Body / Strength / Sports Specific / Health

3 Month Fitness Goals

1 Month Fitness Goals

I plan to exercise ________ days each week.

Before starting any exercise program discuss it with your doctor or medical professional.

My Goals, My Training, and My Success

How am I going to avoid distraction during workout today?

Goal for Today's Workout
Cardiovascular / Weight or Repetitions / Focus / Exercise Form / Other

What did I eat and drink before today's workout?

How do I feel before today's workout?
Energized / Motivated / Content / Drained / Exhausted / Unmotivated

Fitness Journal
My Goals, My Training, and My Success

Strength Exercise Chart	
	Resistance
	Repetitions
	Sets
	Resistance
	Repetitions
	Sets
	Resistance
	Repetitions
	Sets
	Resistance
	Repetitions
	Sets
	Resistance
	Repetitions
	Sets
	Resistance
	Repetitions
	Sets
	Resistance
	Repetitions
	Sets
	Resistance
	Repetitions
	Sets
	Resistance
	Repetitions
	Sets
Cardiovascular Exercise	
	Time
	Time
Stretching Exercise	
	Hold Time
	Hold Time
	Hold Time
	Hold Time

Before starting any exercise program discuss it with your doctor or medical professional.

My Goals, My Training, and My Success

Did I reach my goal for today?________________________

____

____

How do I feel at end of today's workout?
Energized / Motivated / Content / Drained / Exhausted / Disappointed

____

____

____

Goals for next workout:_____________________________

____

____

____

Fitness Trainer's suggestions for next workout:________

____

____

____

Most recent advice from Health Care Professional
Health Status / Goals / Fitness Commitment

____

____

____

____

Were there any injuries or illnesses before or during today's workout?___________________________________

____

____

____

My Goals, My Training, and My Success

Nutritional Section

A great way to discover whether you are getting all of the nutrients your body needs is to write down everything you eat for one week. Once you have the list compare the nutrient values in the foods you have consumed to the nutrient values recommended by your doctor or the recommended dietary allowance. Discuss the results with your doctor or other medical professional in order to improve or maintain your health.

Many people use a chart system similar to this one.

Food	Protein	Vit A	Vit D	Vit E	Vit K	Vit C	Thiamin B1	Riboflavin B2	Niacin B3	Iron	Calcium
Breakfast											
Snack											
Lunch											
Snack											
Dinner											
Snack											
Totals											

Food Consumed Today

Breakfast____

____

Snack____

____

Lunch____

____

____

Snack____
Dinner____

____

____

Snack____

Fitness Journal
My Goals, My Training, and My Success

Motivation for eating healthy:______________________

____

____

____

Immediate nutritional goals:______________________

____

____

____

Did I meet my nutritional goals today?______________

____

____

Long term nutritional or health related goals:________

____

____

____

What changes in nutrition are necessary?
Increase Fluid Intake / Increase Fiber Intake / Decrease Unhealthy Foods /
Decrease Unhealthy Beverages / Increase Fruits or Vegetables / Increase Vitamin
or Mineral____

____

____

____

____

**Recent advice from doctor or other medical professional
regarding nutrition:**______________________________

____

____

____

**Was it difficult to follow the nutritional advice from my
doctor or medical professional?**____________________

____

My Goals, My Training, and My Success

My thoughts:_______________________________

Fitness Journal
My Goals, My Training, and My Success

Fitness Journal 133
My Goals, My Training, and My Success

Name________________________________**Age**_________**Date**___________

Fitness Trainer or Workout Partner_________________________________
Weight_________Percent Body Fat_________Blood Pressure___________
Resting Heart Rate_____________Target Heart Rate____________________
Medications____
____
Medical Problems____
____

Current Fitness Level
Never Exercise / Exercise Occasionally / Weekend Athlete / Exercise
Often / Competitive Athlete / High Fitness Level

____

____

What motivated me to begin a steady exercise program?
Doctor / Health Issues / Upcoming Event / Stress / Social Reasons

____

____

____

Long Term Fitness Goals
Weight Loss / Sculpt Body / Strength / Sports Specific / Health

____

____

____

3 Month Fitness Goals

____

____

____

1 Month Fitness Goals

____

____

____

I plan to exercise _______ days each week.

____

Before starting any exercise program discuss it with your doctor or medical professional.

My Goals, My Training, and My Success

How am I going to avoid distraction during workout today?

____

____

Goal for Today's Workout

Cardiovascular / Weight or Repetitions / Focus / Exercise Form / Other

____

____

____

____

What did I eat and drink before today's workout?

____

____

____

____

How do I feel before today's workout?

Energized / Motivated / Content / Drained / Exhausted / Unmotivated

____

____

My Goals, My Training, and My Success

Strength Exercise Chart		
	Resistance	
	Repetitions	
	Sets	
	Resistance	
	Repetitions	
	Sets	
	Resistance	
	Repetitions	
	Sets	
	Resistance	
	Repetitions	
	Sets	
	Resistance	
	Repetitions	
	Sets	
	Resistance	
	Repetitions	
	Sets	
	Resistance	
	Repetitions	
	Sets	
	Resistance	
	Repetitions	
	Sets	
	Resistance	
	Repetitions	
	Sets	
Cardiovascular Exercise		
	Time	
	Time	
Stretching Exercise		
	Hold Time	
	Hold Time	
	Hold Time	
	Hold Time	

Before starting any exercise program discuss it with your doctor or medical professional.

Fitness Journal
My Goals, My Training, and My Success

Did I reach my goal for today?______________________
____
____

How do I feel at end of today's workout?
Energized / Motivated / Content / Drained / Exhausted / Disappointed
____
____
____

Goals for next workout:______________________
____
____
____

Fitness Trainer's suggestions for next workout:______
____
____
____

Most recent advice from Health Care Professional
Health Status / Goals / Fitness Commitment
____
____
____
____

Were there any injuries or illnesses before or during today's workout?______________________
____
____
____

Before starting any exercise program discuss it with your doctor or medical professional.

My Goals, My Training, and My Success

Nutritional Section

A great way to discover whether you are getting all of the nutrients your body needs is to write down everything you eat for one week. Once you have the list compare the nutrient values in the foods you have consumed to the nutrient values recommended by your doctor or the recommended dietary allowance. Discuss the results with your doctor or other medical professional in order to improve or maintain your health.

Many people use a chart system similar to this one.

Food	Protein	Vit A	Vit D	Vit E	Vit K	Vit C	Thiamin B1	Riboflavin B2	Niacin B3	Iron	Calcium
Breakfast											
Snack											
Lunch											
Snack											
Dinner											
Snack											
Totals											

Food Consumed Today

Breakfast____

____

Snack____

____

Lunch____

____

____

____

Snack____
Dinner____

____

____

Snack____

Fitness Journal
My Goals, My Training, and My Success

Motivation for eating healthy:_______________________

____

____

____

Immediate nutritional goals:_______________________

____

____

____

Did I meet my nutritional goals today?_______________

____

____

Long term nutritional or health related goals:__________

____

____

____

What changes in nutrition are necessary?
Increase Fluid Intake / Increase Fiber Intake / Decrease Unhealthy Foods /
Decrease Unhealthy Beverages / Increase Fruits or Vegetables / Increase Vitamin
or Mineral____

____

____

____

____

**Recent advice from doctor or other medical professional
regarding nutrition:**_______________________________

____

____

____

**Was it difficult to follow the nutritional advice from my
doctor or medical professional?**____________________

____

Before starting any exercise program discuss it with your doctor or medical professional.

My Goals, My Training, and My Success

My thoughts:

Fitness Journal
My Goals, My Training, and My Success

Fitness Journal 141

My Goals, My Training, and My Success

Name_______________________________**Age**________**Date**_________

Fitness Trainer or Workout Partner_________________________________
Weight________Percent Body Fat________Blood Pressure__________
Resting Heart Rate___________Target Heart Rate__________________
Medications____

Medical Problems____
____

Current Fitness Level
Never Exercise / Exercise Occasionally / Weekend Athlete / Exercise
Often / Competitive Athlete / High Fitness Level

____
____

What motivated me to begin a steady exercise program?
Doctor / Health Issues / Upcoming Event / Stress / Social Reasons

____
____
____

Long Term Fitness Goals
Weight Loss / Sculpt Body / Strength / Sports Specific / Health

____
____
____

3 Month Fitness Goals

____
____
____

1 Month Fitness Goals

____
____
____

I plan to exercise ________ days each week.

____

Before starting any exercise program discuss it with your doctor or medical professional.

My Goals, My Training, and My Success

How am I going to avoid distraction during workout today?

____

____

Goal for Today's Workout
Cardiovascular / Weight or Repetitions / Focus / Exercise Form / Other

____

____

____

____

What did I eat and drink before today's workout?

____

____

____

____

How do I feel before today's workout?
Energized / Motivated / Content / Drained / Exhausted / Unmotivated

____

____

My Goals, My Training, and My Success

Strength Exercise Chart		
	Resistance	
	Repetitions	
	Sets	
	Resistance	
	Repetitions	
	Sets	
	Resistance	
	Repetitions	
	Sets	
	Resistance	
	Repetitions	
	Sets	
	Resistance	
	Repetitions	
	Sets	
	Resistance	
	Repetitions	
	Sets	
	Resistance	
	Repetitions	
	Sets	
	Resistance	
	Repetitions	
	Sets	
	Resistance	
	Repetitions	
	Sets	
Cardiovascular Exercise		
	Time	
	Time	
Stretching Exercise		
	Hold Time	
	Hold Time	
	Hold Time	
	Hold Time	

Before starting any exercise program discuss it with your doctor or medical professional.

Fitness Journal
My Goals, My Training, and My Success

Did I reach my goal for today?______________

____

____

How do I feel at end of today's workout?
Energized / Motivated / Content / Drained / Exhausted / Disappointed

Goals for next workout:______________

Fitness Trainer's suggestions for next workout:______

Most recent advice from Health Care Professional
Health Status / Goals / Fitness Commitment

Were there any injuries or illnesses before or during today's workout?______________

My Goals, My Training, and My Success

Nutritional Section

A great way to discover whether you are getting all of the nutrients your body needs is to write down everything you eat for one week. Once you have the list compare the nutrient values in the foods you have consumed to the nutrient values recommended by your doctor or the recommended dietary allowance. Discuss the results with your doctor or other medical professional in order to improve or maintain your health.

Many people use a chart system similar to this one.

Food	Protein	Vit A	Vit D	Vit E	Vit K	Vit C	Thiamin B1	Riboflavin B2	Niacin B3	Iron	Calcium
Breakfast											
Snack											
Lunch											
Snack											
Dinner											
Snack											
Totals											

Food Consumed Today

Breakfast____

____

Snack____

____

Lunch____

____

____

Snack____
Dinner____

____

____

Snack____

Before starting any exercise program discuss it with your doctor or medical professional.

My Goals, My Training, and My Success

Motivation for eating healthy:______________________

____

____

____

Immediate nutritional goals:______________________

____

____

____

Did I meet my nutritional goals today?______________

____

____

Long term nutritional or health related goals:_________

____

____

____

What changes in nutrition are necessary?
Increase Fluid Intake / Increase Fiber Intake / Decrease Unhealthy Foods /
Decrease Unhealthy Beverages / Increase Fruits or Vegetables / Increase Vitamin
or Mineral____

____

____

____

**Recent advice from doctor or other medical professional
regarding nutrition:**___________________________________

____

____

**Was it difficult to follow the nutritional advice from my
doctor or medical professional?**______________________

____

My Goals, My Training, and My Success

My thoughts:____

Fitness Journal
My Goals, My Training, and My Success

My Goals, My Training, and My Success

Name_________________________________**Age**_________**Date**___________

Fitness Trainer or Workout Partner_______________________________
Weight_________Percent Body Fat_________Blood Pressure___________
Resting Heart Rate_____________Target Heart Rate________________
Medications____
____
Medical Problems____
____

Current Fitness Level

Never Exercise / Exercise Occasionally / Weekend Athlete / Exercise
Often / Competitive Athlete / High Fitness Level

____

____

What motivated me to begin a steady exercise program?

Doctor / Health Issues / Upcoming Event / Stress / Social Reasons

____

____

____

Long Term Fitness Goals

Weight Loss / Sculpt Body / Strength / Sports Specific / Health

____

____

____

3 Month Fitness Goals

____

____

____

1 Month Fitness Goals

____

____

____

I plan to exercise _______ days each week.

____

Before starting any exercise program discuss it with your doctor or medical professional.

My Goals, My Training, and My Success

How am I going to avoid distraction during workout today?

____

____

Goal for Today's Workout
Cardiovascular / Weight or Repetitions / Focus / Exercise Form / Other

____

____

____

____

What did I eat and drink before today's workout?

____

____

____

____

How do I feel before today's workout?
Energized / Motivated / Content / Drained / Exhausted / Unmotivated

____

____

My Goals, My Training, and My Success

Strength Exercise Chart	
	Resistance
	Repetitions
	Sets
	Resistance
	Repetitions
	Sets
	Resistance
	Repetitions
	Sets
	Resistance
	Repetitions
	Sets
	Resistance
	Repetitions
	Sets
	Resistance
	Repetitions
	Sets
	Resistance
	Repetitions
	Sets
	Resistance
	Repetitions
	Sets
	Resistance
	Repetitions
	Sets
Cardiovascular Exercise	
	Time
	Time
Stretching Exercise	
	Hold Time
	Hold Time
	Hold Time
	Hold Time

Before starting any exercise program discuss it with your doctor or medical professional.

My Goals, My Training, and My Success

Did I reach my goal for today?________________________

____

____

How do I feel at end of today's workout?
Energized / Motivated / Content / Drained / Exhausted / Disappointed

____

____

____

Goals for next workout:_________________________________

____

____

____

Fitness Trainer's suggestions for next workout:_________

____

____

____

Most recent advice from Health Care Professional
Health Status / Goals / Fitness Commitment

____

____

____

____

Were there any injuries or illnesses before or during today's workout?____

____

____

____

My Goals, My Training, and My Success

Nutritional Section

A great way to discover whether you are getting all of the nutrients your body needs is to write down everything you eat for one week. Once you have the list compare the nutrient values in the foods you have consumed to the nutrient values recommended by your doctor or the recommended dietary allowance. Discuss the results with your doctor or other medical professional in order to improve or maintain your health.

Many people use a chart system similar to this one.

Food	Protein	Vit A	Vit D	Vit E	Vit K	Vit C	Thiamin B1	Riboflavin B2	Niacin B3	Iron	Calcium
Breakfast											
Snack											
Lunch											
Snack											
Dinner											
Snack											
Totals											

Food Consumed Today

Breakfast____

____

Snack____

____

Lunch____

____

____

Snack____
Dinner____

____

____

Snack____

Motivation for eating healthy:_______________________________

____

____

____

Immediate nutritional goals:________________________________

____

____

____

Did I meet my nutritional goals today?_______________________

____

____

Long term nutritional or health related goals:______________

____

____

____

What changes in nutrition are necessary?
Increase Fluid Intake / Increase Fiber Intake / Decrease Unhealthy Foods /
Decrease Unhealthy Beverages / Increase Fruits or Vegetables / Increase Vitamin
or Mineral____

____

____

____

____

**Recent advice from doctor or other medical professional
regarding nutrition:**____

____

____

____

**Was it difficult to follow the nutritional advice from my
doctor or medical professional?**_______________________________

____

My Goals, My Training, and My Success

My thoughts:

My Goals, My Training, and My Success

Fitness Journal
My Goals, My Training, and My Success

Name_______________________________**Age**________**Date**__________

Fitness Trainer or Workout Partner_________________________________
Weight________Percent Body Fat________Blood Pressure__________
Resting Heart Rate___________Target Heart Rate_________________
Medications____
____
Medical Problems____
____

Current Fitness Level
Never Exercise / Exercise Occasionally / Weekend Athlete / Exercise
Often / Competitive Athlete / High Fitness Level

____
____

What motivated me to begin a steady exercise program?
Doctor / Health Issues / Upcoming Event / Stress / Social Reasons

____
____
____

Long Term Fitness Goals
Weight Loss / Sculpt Body / Strength / Sports Specific / Health

____
____
____

3 Month Fitness Goals

____
____
____

1 Month Fitness Goals

____
____
____

I plan to exercise _______ days each week.

____

Before starting any exercise program discuss it with your doctor or medical professional.

My Goals, My Training, and My Success

How am I going to avoid distraction during workout today?

____

____

Goal for Today's Workout

Cardiovascular / Weight or Repetitions / Focus / Exercise Form / Other

____

____

____

____

What did I eat and drink before today's workout?

____

____

____

____

How do I feel before today's workout?

Energized / Motivated / Content / Drained / Exhausted / Unmotivated

____

____

My Goals, My Training, and My Success

Strength Exercise Chart	
	Resistance
	Repetitions
	Sets
	Resistance
	Repetitions
	Sets
	Resistance
	Repetitions
	Sets
	Resistance
	Repetitions
	Sets
	Resistance
	Repetitions
	Sets
	Resistance
	Repetitions
	Sets
	Resistance
	Repetitions
	Sets
	Resistance
	Repetitions
	Sets
	Resistance
	Repetitions
	Sets
Cardiovascular Exercise	
	Time
	Time
Stretching Exercise	
	Hold Time
	Hold Time
	Hold Time
	Hold Time

Before starting any exercise program discuss it with your doctor or medical professional.

Fitness Journal
My Goals, My Training, and My Success

Did I reach my goal for today?________________________

____

____

How do I feel at end of today's workout?
Energized / Motivated / Content / Drained / Exhausted / Disappointed

____

____

____

Goals for next workout:____________________________

____

____

____

Fitness Trainer's suggestions for next workout:________

____

____

____

Most recent advice from Health Care Professional
Health Status / Goals / Fitness Commitment

____

____

____

____

Were there any injuries or illnesses before or during today's workout?_________________________________

____

____

____

My Goals, My Training, and My Success

Nutritional Section

A great way to discover whether you are getting all of the nutrients your body needs is to write down everything you eat for one week. Once you have the list compare the nutrient values in the foods you have consumed to the nutrient values recommended by your doctor or the recommended dietary allowance. Discuss the results with your doctor or other medical professional in order to improve or maintain your health.

Many people use a chart system similar to this one.

Food	Protein	Vit A	Vit D	Vit E	Vit K	Vit C	Thiamin B1	Riboflavin B2	Niacin B3	Iron	Calcium
Breakfast											
Snack											
Lunch											
Snack											
Dinner											
Snack											
Totals											

Food Consumed Today

Breakfast____

____

Snack____

____

Lunch____

____

____

Snack____
Dinner____

____

____

Snack____

My Goals, My Training, and My Success

Motivation for eating healthy:___________________________

____

____

____

Immediate nutritional goals:___________________________

____

____

____

Did I meet my nutritional goals today?_________________

____

____

Long term nutritional or health related goals:__________

____

____

____

What changes in nutrition are necessary?
Increase Fluid Intake / Increase Fiber Intake / Decrease Unhealthy Foods /
Decrease Unhealthy Beverages / Increase Fruits or Vegetables / Increase Vitamin
or Mineral____

____

____

____

____

**Recent advice from doctor or other medical professional
regarding nutrition:**___________________________________

____

____

____

**Was it difficult to follow the nutritional advice from my
doctor or medical professional?**________________________

____

My Goals, My Training, and My Success

My thoughts:_____________________________________

____

My Goals, My Training, and My Success

My Goals, My Training, and My Success

About the Author

Karen Goeller is the author of the famous gymnastics drills and conditioning books. She has been a fitness trainer over 15 years and a gymnastics coach for 25.

Karen's other books include, "Gymnastics Drills and Conditioning for the Handstand" "Over 100 Drills and Conditioning Exercises," "Gymnastics Drills...Walkover, Limber, and Back Handspring," "Gymnastics Conditioning for the Legs and Ankles," "Over 75 Drills and Conditioning Exercises," as well as the book "Gymnastics Journal... My Scores, Mo Goals, My Journal" "The Most Frequently Asked Questions About Gymnastics." She has had gymnastics articles published in Technique Magazine titled, "The Handstand is the Most Important Skill," "Ahh...The Glide Kip" or "Fun with Running, a Crucial Skill".

Before her success as a published author, Karen owned and operated a gymnastics club in NY for 10 years, worked for the most famous gymnastics coach, Bela Karolyi for seven summers, and worked at International Gymnastics Camp for a decade of holiday clinics.

Karen has attended many USA Gymnastics events such as Regional Congress, gymnastics clinics, and the National TOPS Training Camp. Before Karen earned her BA Degree, her studies included Physical Therapy, Health Sciences, and Nutrition. She has held certifications such as a NYS EMT, Nutritional Analysis, Fitness Trainer, and USA Gymnastics Safety among others.

More recently Karen was hired to be a Proctor and Teacher for the Fitness Trainer Certification Exam.

Fitness Journal
My Goals, My Training, and My Success

My Goals, My Training, and My Success

Other Books by this Author

Gymnastics Drills and Conditioning Exercises
ISBN # 1-4116-0579-9
There are over 100 drills and conditioning exercises in this book.
Topics: Running, Vault, Bars, Dance, Press Handstand

Gymnastics Drills and Conditioning for the Handstand
ISBN # 1-4116-5000-X
Topics: Learning Body Tightness, Handstand Shape, Tightness in Motion
and More!

Gymnastics Drills... Walkover, Limber, and Back Handspring
ISBN # 1-4116-1160-8
These drills break down the skills into easy to understand progressions.
The walkover drills can be performed by advanced gymnasts for flexibility.

Gymnastics Conditioning for the Legs and Ankles
ISBN # 1-4116-2033-X
Increase and maintain lower body strength.

Gymnastics Journal... My Scores, My Goals, My Dreams
ISBN # 1-4116-4145-0
It inspires the gymnast to set reasonable goals and track progress.

The Most Frequently Asked Questions about Gymnastics
ISBN # 1-59113-372-6
Guide for gymnastics parents and competitive gymnasts.

www.GymnasticsBooks.com

Before starting any exercise program discuss it with your doctor or medical professional.

My Goals, My Training, and My Success

Warning: Any activity involving exercise, weights, weight machines, or other fitness product creates the possibility of accidental injury, paralysis or death. This journal is intended for use ONLY by healthy adults under medically supervised conditions. Use without proper medical supervision or clearance could be DANGEROUS and should NOT be undertaken or permitted. Before using this journal or beginning any exercise program, KNOW YOUR OWN LIMITATIONS and the limitations of the equipment. If in doubt always consult your health care professional or fitness instructor. When using fitness machines always inspect for loose fittings or damage and ask a trainer to test for stability before each use. We will not be liable for injuries or consequences sustained in the use of this journal, instructional materials, or equipment sold by us.

Although the author of this journal has vast knowledge of health, fitness, and sports in addition to many health related certifications including Fitness Trainer, Nutritional Analysis, and EMT-D, among others, she is not a medical doctor and does not know your personal history.

Before starting any exercise or nutritional program discuss it with your doctor or other medical professional. Always keep safety in mind when performing any exercise and when making changes in your eating habits.

We wish you the best of luck in reaching your health and fitness goals!

www.ingramcontent.com/pod-product-compliance
Lightning Source LLC
Chambersburg PA
CBHW051450250726
48655CB00001B/346